The Air Fryer Healthy Cooking Guide

Discover the Pleasures of Air Fryer Meals with These Amazing Recipes

Franck McMillan

TABLE OF CONTENT

Crunchy Parmesan Asparagus 7
Bacon Bell Peppers 9
Corn & Carrot Fritters 10
Butter Baked Nuts 12
Eggs Spinach Side 15
Squash and Cumin Chili 17
Fried Up Avocados 19
Hearty Green Beans 20
Parmesan Cabbage Wedges 21
Extreme Zucchini Fries 22
Easy Fried Tomatoes 24
Roasted Up Brussels 26
Roasted Brussels and Pine Nuts 28
Low-Calorie Beets Dish 30
Broccoli and Parmesan Dish 31
Bacon and Asparagus Spears 32
Healthy Low Carb Fish Nugget 33
Fried Up Pumpkin Seeds 35
Decisive Tiger Shrimp Platter 37
Air Fried Olives 39
Bacon-Wrapped Dates 41
Bacon-Wrapped Shrimp and Jalapeño 43

Breaded Artichoke Hearts 45
Bruschetta with Basil Pesto 47
Cajun Zucchini Chips 49
Cheesy Apple Roll-Ups 51
Cheesy Jalapeño Poppers 53
Cheesy Steak Fries 55
Crispy Breaded Beef Cubes 57
Coriander Artichokes 59
Spinach and Artichokes Sauté 60
Green Beans 61
Turmeric Mushroom 63
Creamy Fennel 64
Air Fried Green Tomatoes 65
Seasoned Potato Wedges 67
Honey Roasted Carrots 69
Onion Rings 70
Chicken Kebab 72
Cinnamon Apple Chips 74
Apple Chips with Dip 75
Delicious Spiced Apples 76
Tasty Cheese Bites 77
Apple Chips 79
Gooey Cinnamon Smores 80
Sweetened Plantains 82
Pear Crisp 83

Easy Pears Dessert *84*
Vanilla Strawberry Mix *85*
Sweet Bananas and Sauce *86*
Cinnamon Apples and Mandarin Sauce *87*
Cocoa Berries Cream *88*
Sweet Vanilla Rhubarb *89*
Cherries and Rhubarb Bowls *90*
Pumpkin Bowls *91*
Buttery Fennel and Garlic *92*
Lemon Mousse *94*
Glazed Banana *96*
Raspberry Danish *98*
Blueberry Muffins *101*
Cranberry Cupcakes *104*
Zucchini Mug Cake *106*
Chocolate Brownies *108*
Apple Crisp *110*

© Copyright 2021 - All rights reserved.

The content contained within this book may not be reproduced, duplicated or transmitted without direct written permission from the author or the publisher.

Under no circumstances will any blame or legal responsibility be held against the publisher, or author, for any damages, reparation, or monetary loss due to the information contained within this book. Either directly or indirectly.

Legal Notice:

This book is copyright protected. This book is only for personal use. You cannot amend, distribute, sell, use, quote or paraphrase any part, or the content within this book, without the consent of the author or publisher.

Disclaimer Notice:

Please note the information contained within this document is for educational and entertainment purposes only. All effort has been executed to present accurate, up to date, and reliable, complete information. No warranties of any kind are declared or implied. Readers acknowledge that the author is not engaging in the rendering of legal, financial, medical or professional advice. The content within this book has been derived from various sources. Please consult a licensed professional before attempting any techniques outlined in this book.

By reading this document, the reader agrees that under no circumstances is the author responsible for any losses, direct or indirect, which are incurred as a result of the use of information contained within this document, including, but not limited to, — errors, omissions, or inaccuracies.

Crunchy Parmesan Asparagus

Preparation Time: 10 Minutes

Cooking Time: 10 Minutes

Servings: 4

Ingredients:

- 1/4 cup all-purpose flour
- Salt to taste
- 2 eggs, beaten
- 1/4 cup Parmesan cheese, grated
- 1/2 cup breadcrumbs
- 1 cup asparagus, trimmed
- Cooking spray

Directions:

1. Mix flour and salt in a bowl.
2. Add eggs to a second bowl.
3. Combine Parmesan cheese and breadcrumbs in a third bowl.
4. Dip asparagus spears in the first, second and third bowls.
5. Spray with oil.

6. Add crisper plate to the air fryer basket inside the Power XL Grill.
7. Set it to air fry.
8. Preheat at 390 degrees F for 3 minutes.
9. Add asparagus to the plate.
10. Air fry for 5 minutes per side.

Nutrition: Calories: 243 Fat: 10.5g Saturated Fat: 3g Trans Fat: 0g Carbohydrates: 10g Fiber: 3g Sodium: 824mg Protein: 35g

Bacon Bell Peppers

Preparation Time: 10 Minutes

Cooking Time: 5 Minutes

Servings: 16

Ingredients:

- 1 pack bacon slices
- 12 bell peppers, sliced in half
- 8 oz. cream cheese

Directions:

1. Stuff bell pepper halves with cream cheese.
2. Wrap with bacon slices.
3. Preheat Power XL Grill to 500 degrees F.
4. Add bell peppers to the grill.
5. Grill for 3 to 5 minutes.

Nutrition: Calories - 482 Fat – 42g Carbohydrates – 14g Fiber – 5g Protein – 28g

Corn & Carrot Fritters

Preparation Time: 8 to 10 Minutes

Cooking Time: 12 Minutes

Servings: 4 to 5

Ingredients:

- 4 ounces canned sweet corn kernels, drained
- 1 teaspoon sea salt flakes
- 1 tablespoon cilantro, chopped
- 1 carrot, grated
- 1 yellow onion, finely chopped
- 1 medium-sized egg, whisked
- 1/4 cup of self-rising flour
- 1/3 teaspoon baking powder
- 2 tablespoons milk
- 1 cup Parmesan cheese, grated
- 1/3 teaspoon brown sugar

Directions:

1. Place your air fryer on a flat kitchen surface; plug it and turn it on. Set temperature to 350 degrees F and let it preheat for 4-5 minutes.

2. Press the carrot in the colander to remove excess liquid. Arrange the carrot between several sheets of kitchen towels and pat it dry.
3. Then, mix the carrots with the remaining ingredients in a big bowl. Make small balls from the mixture.
4. Gently flatten them with your hand. Spitz the balls with a nonstick cooking oil.
5. Add the in balls the basket.
6. Push the air-frying basket in the air fryer. Cook for 8-10 minutes.
7. Slide out the basket; serve warm!

Nutrition: Calories - 274 Fat – 8.3g Carbohydrates – 38.8g Fiber – 2.3g Protein – 15.6g

Butter Baked Nuts

Preparation Time: 10 Minutes

Cooking Time: 15 Minutes

Servings: 4

Ingredients:

- 1 cup raw almonds or pistachios
- 1 cup raw peanuts
- 1 tablespoon butter, melted
- ½ cup raw cashew nuts
- Salt to taste

Directions:

1. Take Power XL multi-cooker, arrange it over a cooking platform, and open the top lid.
2. In the pot, arrange a reversible rack and place the Crisping Basket over the rack.
3. In the basket, add the nuts.
4. Seal the multi-cooker by locking it with the crisping lid; ensure to keep the pressure release valve locked/sealed.
5. Select the "AIR CRISP" mode and adjust the 350°F temperature level. Then, set Timer to 10 minutes and press "STOP/START"; it

will start the cooking process by building up inside pressure.
6. When the Timer goes off, quick release pressure by adjusting the pressure valve to the VENT.
7. After pressure gets released, open the pressure lid.
8. Add the butter on top and season with some salt; shake well.
9. Seal the multi-cooker by locking it with the crisping lid; ensure to keep the pressure release valve locked/sealed.
10. Select "BAKE/ROAST" mode and adjust the 350°F temperature level. Then, set Timer to 5 minutes and press "STOP/START"; it will start the cooking process by building up inside pressure.
11. When the Timer goes off, quick release pressure by adjusting the pressure valve to the VENT. After pressure gets released, open the pressure lid.
12. Serve warm and enjoy!

Nutrition: Calories: 192 Fat: 16g Saturated Fat: 2g Trans Fat: 0g Carbohydrates: 6.5g Fiber: 3g Sodium:

64mg Protein: 7.5g

Eggs Spinach Side

Preparation Time: 5 Minutes

Cooking Time: 12 Minutes

Servings: 2 to 3

Ingredients:

- 1 medium-sized tomato, chopped
- 1 teaspoon lemon juice
- 1/2 teaspoon coarse salt
- 2 tablespoons olive oil
- 4 eggs, whisked
- 5 ounces spinach, chopped
- 1/2 teaspoon black pepper
- 1/2 cup basil, roughly chopped

Directions:

1. Place your air fryer on a flat kitchen surface; plug it and turn it on. Set temperature to 280 degrees F and let it preheat for 4-5 minutes.
2. Take out the air-frying basket and gently coat it using the olive oil.
3. In a bowl of medium size, thoroughly mix the ingredients except for the basil leaves.

4. Add the mixture to the basket. Push the air-frying basket in the air fryer. Cook for 10-12 minutes.
5. Slide out the basket; top with basil and serve warm with sour cream!

Nutrition: Calories – 272 Fat, – 23g Carbohydrates – 5.4g Fiber – 2g Protein – 13.2g

Squash and Cumin Chili

Preparation Time: 10 Minutes

Cooking Time: 16 Minutes

Servings: 4

Ingredients:

- One medium butternut squash
- One teaspoon cumin seed
- One large pinch of chili flakes
- One tablespoon olive oil
- One and ½ ounces pine nuts
- One small bunch of fresh coriander, chopped

Directions:

1. Take the squash and slice it
2. Remove seeds and cut into smaller chunks
3. Take a bowl and add chunked squash, spice, and oil
4. Mix well
5. Pre-heat your Fryer to 360 degrees F and add the squash to the cooking basket
6. Roast for 20 minutes. Ensure to shake the basket from Time to Time to avoid burning

7. Take a pan and place it over medium heat, add pine nuts to the pan, and dry toast for 2 minutes
8. Sprinkle nuts on top of the squash and serve
9. Enjoy!

Nutrition: Calories: 414 Fat: 15g Carbohydrates: 10g Protein: 16g

Fried Up Avocados

Preparation Time: 10 Minutes

Cooking Time: 20 Minutes

Servings: 6

Ingredients:

- ½ cup almond meal
- ½ teaspoon salt
- 1 Hass avocado, peeled, pitted, and sliced
- Aquafaba from one bean can (bean liquid)

Directions:

1. Take a shallow bowl and add almond meal, salt
2. Pour aquafaba in another bowl, dredge avocado slices in aquafaba and then into the crumbs to get a nice coating
3. Assemble them in a single layer in your Air Fryer cooking basket, don't overlap
4. Cook for 10 minutes at 390 degrees F, give the basket a shake, and cook for 5 minutes more
5. Serve and enjoy!

Nutrition: Calories: 356 Fat: 14g Carbohydrates: 8g Protein: 23g

Hearty Green Beans

Preparation Time: 5 Minutes

Cooking Time: 10 to 15 Minutes

Servings: 6

Ingredients:

- 1-pound green beans washed and de-stemmed
- One lemon
- Pinch of salt
- ¼ teaspoon oil

Directions:

1. Add beans to your Air Fryer cooking basket
2. Squeeze a few drops of lemon
3. Season with salt and pepper
4. Drizzle olive oil on top
5. Cook for 10-12 minutes at 400 degrees F
6. Once done, serve and enjoy!

Nutrition: Calories: 84 Fat: 5g Carbohydrates: 7g Protein: 2g

Parmesan Cabbage Wedges

Preparation Time: 5 Minutes

Cooking Time: 20 Minutes

Servings: 4

Ingredients:

- ½ a head cabbage
- 2 cups parmesan
- Four tablespoons melted butter
- Salt and pepper to taste

Directions:

1. Preheat your Air Fryer to 380-degree F.
2. Take a container and add melted butter, and season with salt and pepper.
3. Cover cabbages with your melted butter.
4. Coat cabbages with parmesan.
5. Transfer the coated cabbages to your Air Fryer and bake for 20 minutes.
6. Serve with cheesy sauce and enjoy!

Nutrition: Calories: 108 Fat: 7g Carbohydrates: 11g Protein: 2g

Extreme Zucchini Fries

Preparation Time: 10 Minutes

Cooking Time: 15 to 20 Minutes

Servings: 4

Ingredients:
1. Three medium zucchinis, sliced
2. Two egg whites
3. ½ cup seasoned almond meal
4. Two tablespoons grated parmesan cheese
5. ¼ teaspoon garlic powder

Directions:
1. Pre-heat your Fryer to 425-degree F.
2. Take the Air Fryer cooking basket and place a cooling rack.
3. Coat the rack with cooking spray.
4. Take a bowl, add egg whites, beat it well, and season with some pepper and salt.
5. Take another bowl and add garlic powder, cheese, and almond meal
6. Take the Zucchini sticks and dredge them in the egg and finally breadcrumbs.
7. Transfer the Zucchini to your cooking basket and spray a bit of oil.

8. Bake for 20 minutes and serve with Ranch sauce.
9. Enjoy!

Nutrition: Calories: 367 Fat: 28g Carbohydrates: 5g Protein: 4g

Easy Fried Tomatoes

Preparation Time: 5 Minutes

Cooking Time: 10 Minutes

Servings: 3

Ingredients:

- One green tomato
- ¼ tablespoon Creole seasoning
- Salt and pepper to taste
- ¼ cup almond flour
- ½ cup buttermilk

Directions:

1. Add flour to your plate and take another plate and add buttermilk
2. Cut tomatoes and season with salt and pepper
3. Make a mix of creole seasoning and crumbs
4. Take tomato slice and cover with flour, place in buttermilk and then into crumbs
5. Repeat with all tomatoes
6. Preheat your fryer to 400-degree F
7. Cook the tomato slices for 5 minutes
8. Serve with basil and enjoy!

Nutrition: Calories: 166 Fat: 12g Carbohydrates: 11g Protein: 3g

Roasted Up Brussels

Preparation Time: 10 Minutes

Cooking Time: 15 Minutes

Servings: 4

Ingredients:

- One block Brussels sprouts
- ½ teaspoon garlic
- Two teaspoons olive oil
- ½ teaspoon pepper
- Salt as needed

Directions:

1. Pre-heat your Fryer to 390-degree F.
2. Remove leaves off the chokes, leaving only the head.
3. Wash and dry the sprouts well.
4. Make a mixture of olive oil, salt, and pepper with garlic.
5. Cover sprouts with the marinade and let them rest for 5 minutes.
6. Transfer coated sprouts to Air Fryer and cook for 15 minutes.
7. Serve and enjoy!

Nutrition: Calories: 43 Fat: 2g Carbohydrates: 5g

Protein: 2g

Roasted Brussels and Pine Nuts

Preparation Time: 10 Minutes

Cooking Time: 35 Minutes

Servings: 6

Ingredients:

- 15 ounces Brussels sprouts
- One tablespoon olive oil
- One and ¾ ounces raisins, drained
- Juice of 1 orange
- One and ¾ ounces toasted pine nuts

Directions:

1. Take a pot of boiling water, then add sprouts and boil them for 4 minutes.
2. Transfer the sprouts to cold water and drain them well.
3. Place them in a freezer and cool them.
4. Take your raisins and soak them in orange juice for 20 minutes.
5. Warm your Air Fryer to a temperature of 392-degree F.
6. Take a pan and pour oil, and stir the sprouts.

7. Take the sprouts and transfer them to your Air Fryer.
8. Roast for 15 minutes.
9. Serve the sprouts with pine nuts, orange juice, and raisins!

Nutrition: Calories: 260 Fat: 20g Carbohydrates: 10g Protein: 7g

Low-Calorie Beets Dish

Preparation Time: 10 Minutes

Cooking Time: 10 Minutes

Servings: 2

Ingredients:

- Four whole beets
- One tablespoon balsamic vinegar
- One tablespoon olive oil
- Salt and pepper to taste
- Two springs rosemary

Directions:

1. Wash your beets and peel them
2. Cut beets into cubes
3. Take a bowl and mix in rosemary, pepper, salt, vinegar
4. Cover beets with the sauce
5. Coat the beets with olive oil
6. Pre-heat your Fryer to 400-degree F
7. Transfer beets to Air Fryer cooking basket and cook for 10 minutes
8. Serve with your cheese sauce and enjoy!

Nutrition: Calories: 149 Fat: 1g Carbohydrates: 5g Protein: 30g

Broccoli and Parmesan Dish

Preparation Time: 5 Minutes

Cooking Time: 20 Minutes

Servings: 4

Ingredients:

- One fresh head broccoli
- One tablespoon olive oil
- One lemon, juiced
- Salt and pepper to taste
- 1-ounce parmesan cheese, grated

Directions:

1. Wash broccoli thoroughly and cut them into florets.
2. Add the listed Ingredients: to your broccoli and mix well.
3. Preheat your fryer to 365-degree F.
4. Air fry broccoli for 20 minutes.
5. Serve and enjoy!

Nutrition: Calories: 114 Fat: 6g Carbohydrates: 10 g Protein: 7g

Bacon and Asparagus Spears

Preparation Time: 15 Minutes

Cooking Time: 8 Minutes

Servings: 4

Ingredients:

- 20 spears asparagus
- Four bacon slices
- One tablespoon olive oil
- One tablespoon sesame oil
- One garlic clove, crushed

Directions:

1. Warm your Air Fryer to 380 degrees F
2. Take a small bowl and add oil, crushed garlic, and mix
3. Separate asparagus into four bunches and wrap them in bacon
4. Brush wraps with oil and garlic mix, transfer to your Air Fryer basket
5. Cook for 8 minutes
6. Serve and enjoy!

Nutrition: Calories: 175 Fat: 15g Carbohydrates: 6g Protein: 5g

Healthy Low Carb Fish Nugget

Preparation Time: 5 Minutes

Cooking Time: 10 Minutes

Servings: 4

Ingredients:

- 1-pound fresh cod
- Two tablespoons olive oil
- ½ cup almond flour
- Two larges finely beaten eggs
- 1-2 cups almond meal

Directions:

1. Preheat your Air Fryer to 388 degrees F
2. Take a food processor and add olive oil, almond meal, salt, and blend
3. Take three bowls and add almond flour, almond meal, beaten eggs individually
4. Take cods and cut them into slices of 1-inch thickness and 2-inch length
5. Dredge slices into flour, eggs, and crumbs
6. Transfer nuggets to Air Fryer cooking basket and cook for 10 minutes until golden

7. Serve and enjoy!

Nutrition: Calories: 196 Fat: 14g Carbohydrates: 6g Protein: 14g

Fried Up Pumpkin Seeds

Preparation Time: 10 Minutes

Cooking Time: 60 Minutes

Servings: 2

Ingredients:

- One and ½ cups pumpkin seeds
- Olive oil as needed
- One and ½ teaspoons salt
- One teaspoon smoked paprika

Directions:

1. Cut pumpkin and scrape out seeds and flesh
2. Separate flesh from seeds and rinse the seeds under cold water
3. Bring two-quarter of salted water to boil and add seeds, boil for 10 minutes
4. Drain seeds and spread them on a kitchen towel
5. Dry for 20 minutes
6. Preheat your fryer to 350 degrees F
7. Take a bowl and add seeds, smoked paprika, and olive oil

8. Season with salt and transfer to your Air Fryer cooking basket
9. Cook for 35 minutes, enjoy it!

Nutrition: Calories: 237 Fat: 21g Carbohydrates: 4g Protein: 12g

Decisive Tiger Shrimp Platter

Preparation Time: 5 Minutes

Cooking Time: 10 Minutes

Servings: 6

Ingredients:

- One ¼ pound tiger shrimp, or a count of about 16 to 20
- ¼ teaspoons cayenne pepper
- ½ teaspoons old bay seasoning
- ¼ teaspoons smoked paprika
- One tablespoon olive oil

Directions:

1. Pre-heat your Fryer to 390-degree Fahrenheit
2. Take a bowl and add the listed Ingredients:
3. Mix well
4. Transfer the shrimp to your fryer cooking basket and cook for 5 minutes
5. Remove and serve the shrimp over cauliflower rice if preferred
6. Enjoy!

Nutrition: Calories: 251 Carbohydrate: 3g Protein:

17g Fat: 19g

Air Fried Olives

Preparation Time: 5 Minutes

Cooking Time: 8 Minutes

Servings: 4

Ingredients:

- 1 (5½-ounce / 156-g) jar pitted green olives
- ½ cup all-purpose flour
- Salt and pepper, to taste
- ½ cup bread crumbs
- One egg

Directions:

1. Preheat the air fryer oven to 400°F (204°C).
2. Take away the olives from the jar and dry thoroughly with paper towels.
3. In a small bowl, combine the flour with salt and pepper to taste. Place the bread crumbs in another small container. In a third small bowl, beat the egg.
4. Spray the basket with cooking spray.
5. Drench the olives in the flour, then the egg, and then the bread crumbs.

6. Place the breaded olives in the air fryer basket. It is okay to stack them. Spray the olives with cooking spray.
7. Place the air fryer basket onto the warming pan.
8. Slide into Rack Position 2.
9. Select Air Fry and set the Time to 6 minutes.
10. Flip the olives and air fry for an additional 2 minutes, or until brown and crisp.
11. Cool for 5 minutes before serving.

Nutrition: Calories: 188 Fat: 6.8g Carbs: 1.9g Protein: 30.3g

Bacon-Wrapped Dates

Preparation Time: 10 Minutes

Cooking Time: 6 Minutes

Servings: 6

Ingredients:

- 12 dates, pitted
- Six slices of high-quality bacon, cut in half
- Cooking spray

Directions:

1. Preheat the air fryer oven to 360°F (182°C).
2. Covering each date with half a bacon slice and secure with a toothpick.
3. Spray the air fryer basket by means of cooking spray, then place bacon-wrapped dates in the basket.
4. Place the air fryer basket onto the baking pan.
5. Slide into Rack Position 2, select Air Fry, set Time to 6 minutes, or wait until the bacon is crispy.
6. Remove the dates and allow them to cool on a wire rack for 5 minutes before serving.

Nutrition: Calories: 246 Protein: 14.4g Fiber: 0.6 g Net Carbohydrates: 2.0 g Fat: 17.9 g Sodium: 625 Mg Carbohydrates: 2.6 g

Bacon-Wrapped Shrimp and Jalapeño

Preparation Time: 20 Minutes

Cooking Time: 13 Minutes

Servings: 8

Ingredients:

- 24 large shrimp, peeled and deveined, about ¾ pound (340 g)
- Five tablespoons barbecue sauce, divided
- 12 strips bacon, cut in half
- 24 small pickled jalapeño slices

Directions:

1. Toss together the shrimp and three tablespoons of the barbecue sauce. Let stand for 15 minutes. Soak 24 wooden toothpicks in water for 10 minutes. Wrap 1-piece bacon around the shrimp and jalapeño slice, then secure with a toothpick.
2. Preheat the air fryer oven to 350°F (177°C).
3. Position the shrimp in the air fryer basket, spacing them ½ inch apart.

4. Place the air fryer basket onto the baking pan.
5. Slide into Rack Position 2, select Air Fry, and set Time to 10 minutes.
6. Turn shrimp over with tongs and air fry for 3 minutes more, or until bacon is golden brown and shrimp are cooked through.
7. Brush with the remaining barbecue sauce and serve.

Nutrition: Calories: 246 Protein: 14.4g Fiber: 0.6 g Net Carbohydrates: 2.0 g Fat: 17.9 g Sodium: 625 Mg Carbohydrates: 2.6 g

Breaded Artichoke Hearts

Preparation Time: 5 Minutes

Cooking Time: 8 Minutes

Servings: 14

Ingredients:

- 14 whole artichoke hearts, packed in water
- One egg
- ½ cup all-purpose flour
- 1/3 cup panko bread crumbs
- One teaspoon Italian seasoning

Directions:

1. Preheat the air fryer oven to 380ºF (193ºC)
2. Squeeze excess water from the artichoke hearts and place them on paper towels to dry.
3. In a small bowl, beat the egg.
4. In another small bowl, place the flour.
5. In a third small bowl, blend the bread crumbs and Italian seasoning, and stir.
6. Spritz the air fryer basket by means of cooking spray.

7. Drench the artichoke hearts in the flour, then the egg, and then the bread crumb mixture.
8. Place the breaded artichoke hearts in the air fryer basket. Spray them with cooking spray.
9. Place the air fryer basket onto the baking pan.
10. Slide into Rack Position 2, select Air Fry, and set Time to 8 minutes. You may wait until the artichoke hearts have browned and are crisp. Flip once halfway through the cooking Time.
11. Let cool for 5 minutes before serving.

Nutrition: Calories: 149 Fat: 1g Carbohydrates: 5g Protein: 30g

Bruschetta with Basil Pesto

Preparation Time: 10 Minutes

Cooking Time: 5 to 7 Minutes

Servings: 4

Ingredients:

- Eight slices French bread, ½ inch thick
- Two tablespoons softened butter
- 1 cup shredded Mozzarella cheese
- ½ cup basil pesto
- 1 cup chopped grape tomatoes

Directions:

1. Preheat the air fryer oven to 350ºF (177ºC).
2. Spread the bread with the butter and position butter-side up in a baking pan.
3. Slide the baking pan into Rack Position 1, select Convection Bake, set Time to 4 minutes, or wait until the bread is light golden brown.
4. Remove the bread from the oven and top each piece with some of the cheese.

5. Back to the oven and bake for 1 to 3 minutes more, or until the cheese melts.
6. In the meantime, combine the pesto, tomatoes, and green onions in a small bowl.
7. When the cheese has melted, take away the oven's bread and put on a serving platter. Top each slice utilizing some of the pesto mixtures and serve.

Nutrition: Calories: 251 Carbohydrate: 3g Protein: 17g Fat: 19g

Cajun Zucchini Chips

Preparation Time: 5 Minutes

Cooking Time: 16 Minutes

Servings: 4

Ingredients:

- Two large zucchinis, cut into 1/8-inch-thick slices
- Two teaspoons Cajun seasoning
- Cooking spray

Directions:

1. Preheat the air fryer oven to 370°F (188°C).
2. Spray the air fryer basket lightly with cooking spray.
3. Put the zucchini slices in a medium bowl and spray them generously with cooking spray.
4. Sprinkle the Cajun seasoning over the zucchini and stir to make sure they are evenly coated with oil and seasoning.
5. Position the slices in a single layer in the air fryer basket, making sure not to overcrowd.

6. Place the air fryer basket onto the baking pan.
7. Slide into Rack Position 2
8. Select Air Fry and set the Time to 8 minutes.
9. Flip the slices over and air fry for an additional 7 to 8 minutes, or until they are as crunchy and brown as you prefer.
10. Serve immediately.

Nutrition: Calories: 367 Fat: 28g Carbohydrates: 5g Protein: 4g

Cheesy Apple Roll-Ups

Preparation Time: 5 Minutes

Cooking Time: 5 Minutes

Servings: 8

Ingredients:

1. Eight slices whole wheat sandwich bread
2. 4 ounces (113 g) Colby Jack cheese, grated
3. ½ small apple, chopped
4. Two tablespoons butter, melted

Directions:

1. Preheat the air fryer oven to 390°F (199°C).
2. Take away the crusts from the bread and flatten the slices with a rolling pin. Don't be gentle. Press hard so that the bread will be fragile.
3. Top bread slices with cheese and chopped apple, dividing the Ingredients: evenly.
4. Roll up each slice tightly and secure each with one or two toothpicks.
5. Brush outside of rolls with melted butter. Place them in the air fryer basket.

6. Place the air fryer basket onto the baking pan.
7. Slide into Rack Position 2, select Air Fry, and set Time to 5 minutes. You may also wait until the outside is crisp and nicely browned.
8. Serve hot.

Nutrition: Calories: 147 Fat: 9.5g Carbohydrates: 13.8g Sugar: 2.1g Protein: 1.9g Sodium: 62mg

Cheesy Jalapeño Poppers

Preparation Time: 5 Minutes

Cooking Time: 10 Minutes

Servings: 4

Ingredients:

- Eight jalapeño peppers
- ½ cup whipped cream cheese
- ¼ cup shredded Cheddar cheese

Directions:

1. Preheat the air fryer oven to 360ºF (182ºC).
2. Practice a paring knife to carefully cut off the jalapeño tops, then scoop out the ribs and seeds. Set aside.
3. In a medium bowl, combine the whipped cream cheese and shredded Cheddar cheese. Place the mixture in a sealable plastic bag, and using a pair of scissors, cut off one corner from the bag. Gently squeeze some cream cheese mixture into each pepper until almost full.

4. Place a piece of parchment paper on the bottom of the air fryer basket and place the poppers on top, distributing evenly.
5. Place the air fryer basket onto the baking pan.
6. Slide into Rack Position 2, select Air Fry, and set Time to 10 minutes.
7. Allow the poppers to cool for 5 to 10 minutes before serving.

Nutrition: Calories: 456 Fat: 60g Carbohydrates: 7g Protein: 15g

Cheesy Steak Fries

Preparation Time: 5 Minutes

Cooking Time: 20 Minutes

Servings: 5

Ingredients:

- 1 (28-ounce / 794-g) bag frozen steak fries
- Cooking spray
- ½ cup beef gravy
- 1 cup shredded Mozzarella cheese
- Two scallions, green parts only, chopped

Directions:

1. Preheat the air fryer oven to 400°F (204°C).
2. Place the frozen steak fries in the air fryer basket.
3. Place the air fryer basket onto the baking pan.
4. Slide into Rack Position 2, select Air Fry, and set Time to 10 minutes.
5. Shake the basket and spritz the fries with cooking spray. Sprinkle with salt and pepper. Air fry for an additional 8 minutes.

6. Pour the beef gravy into a medium, microwave-safe bowl—microwave for 30 seconds, or until the sauce is warm.
7. Sprinkle the fries with the cheese. Air fry for an additional 2 minutes until the cheese is melted.
8. Transfer the fries to a serving dish. Drizzle the fries with gravy and sprinkle the scallions on top for a green garnish. Serve warm.

Nutrition: Calories 1536Fat 123.7g Protein 103.4 g

Crispy Breaded Beef Cubes

Preparation Time: 10 Minutes

Cooking Time: 8 Minutes

Servings: 4

Ingredients:

- 1-pound (454 g) sirloin tip, cut into 1-inch cubes
- 1 cup cheese pasta sauce
- 1½ cups soft bread crumbs
- Two tablespoons olive oil
- ½ teaspoon dried marjoram

Directions:

1. Preheat the air fryer oven to 360°F (182°C).
2. In a medium container, toss the beef with the pasta sauce to coat.
3. In a shallow bowl, blend the bread crumbs, oil, and marjoram, and stir completely. Put the beef cubes, one at a Time, into the bread crumb mixture to coat methodically. Transfer the beef to the air fryer basket.
4. Place the air fryer basket onto the baking pan.

5. Slide into Rack Position 2, select Air Fry, set Time to 8 minutes, or until the beef is at least 145ºF (63ºC), and the outside is crisp and brown. Shake the basket once during cooking Time.
6. Serve hot.

Nutrition: Calories: 262 kcal Total Fat: 9.4g Carbs: 8.2g Protein: 16.2g

Coriander Artichokes

Preparation Time: 5 Minutes

Cooking Time: 20 Minutes

Servings: 4

Ingredients:
1. 12 oz. artichoke hearts
2. 1 tbsp. lemon juice
3. 1 tsp. coriander, ground
4. ½ tsp. cumin seeds
5. ½ tsp. olive oil

Directions:
1. Mix all the ingredients, toss.
2. Introduce the pan in the fryer and cook at 370°F for 15 minutes
3. Divide the mix between plates and serve as a side dish.

Nutrition: Calories: 200 Fat: 7g Fiber: 2g Carbs: 5g Protein: 8g

Spinach and Artichokes Sauté

Preparation Time: 5 Minutes

Cooking Time: 20 Minutes

Servings: 4

Ingredients:

- 10 oz. artichoke hearts; halved
- 2 cups baby spinach
- Three garlic cloves
- ¼ cup veggie stock
- 2 tsp. lime juice
- Salt and black pepper to taste.

Directions:

1. Mix all the ingredients, toss, introduce in the fryer and cook at 370°F for 15 minutes
2. Divide between plates and serve.

Nutrition: Calories: 209 Fat: 6g Fiber: 2g Carbs: 4g Protein: 8g

Green Beans

Preparation Time: 5 Minutes

Cooking Time: 25 Minutes

Servings: 4

Ingredients:

- 6 cups green beans; trimmed
- 1 tbsp. hot paprika
- 2 tbsp. olive oil
- A pinch of salt and black pepper

Directions:

1. Take a bowl and mix the green beans with the other ingredients, toss, put them in the air fryer's basket and cook at 370°F for 20 minutes
2. Divide among plates and serve as a side dish.

Nutrition: Calories: 120 Fat: 5g Fiber: 1g Carbs: 4g Protein: 2g

Bok Choy and Butter Sauce

Preparation Time: 5 Minutes

Cooking Time: 20 Minutes

Servings: 4

Ingredients:

- Two bok choy heads; trimmed and cut into strips
- 1 tbsp. butter; melted
- 2 tbsp. chicken stock
- 1 tsp. lemon juice
- 1 tbsp. olive oil

Directions:

1. Mix all the ingredients, toss, introduce the pan to the air fryer, then cook at 380°F for 15 minutes.
2. Split between plates and serve as a side dish

Nutrition: Calories: 141 Fat: 3g Fiber: 2g Carbs: 4g Protein: 3g

Turmeric Mushroom

Preparation Time: 5 Minutes

Cooking Time: 20 Minutes

Servings: 4

Ingredients:

- 1 lb. brown mushrooms
- Four garlic cloves; minced
- ¼ tsp. cinnamon powder
- 1 tsp. olive oil
- ½ tsp. turmeric powder

Directions:

1. Mix all the fixings and toss.
2. Put the mushrooms in your air fryer's basket and cook at 370°F for 15 minutes
3. Divide the mix between plates and serve as a side dish.

Nutrition: Calories: 208 Fat: 7g Fiber: 3g Carbs: 5g Protein: 7g

Creamy Fennel

Preparation Time:5 Minutes

Cooking Time: 17 Minutes

Servings: 4

Ingredients:

- Two big fennel bulbs; sliced
- ½ cup coconut cream
- 2 tbsp. butter; melted
- Salt and black pepper to taste.

Directions:

1. In a pan that fits the air fryer, combine all the ingredients, toss, introduce in the machine and cook at 370°F for 12 minutes
2. Divide between plates and serve as a side dish.

Nutrition: Calories: 151 Fat: 3g Fiber: 2g Carbs: 4g Protein: 6g

Air Fried Green Tomatoes

Preparation Time: 5 Minutes

Cooking Time: 17 Minutes

Servings: 4

Ingredients:

- Two medium green tomatoes
- 1/3 cup grated Parmesan cheese.
- ¼ cup blanched finely ground almond flour.
- One large egg.

Directions:

1. Slice tomatoes into ½-inch-thick slices. Take a medium bowl, whisk the egg. Take a large bowl, mix the almond flour and Parmesan.
2. Dip each tomato slice into the egg, then scour in the almond flour mixture. Position the slices into the air fryer basket
3. Adjust the temperature to 400 Degrees F and set the Timer for 7 minutes. Flip the slices midway over the cooking Time. Serve immediately

Nutrition: Calories: 106 Protein: 6.2g Fiber: 1.4g Fat:

6.7g Carbs: 5.9g

Seasoned Potato Wedges

Preparation Time: 10 Minutes

Cooking Time: 20 Minutes

Servings: 4

Ingredients:

- Four russet potatoes
- One tablespoon bacon fat
- One teaspoon paprika
- One teaspoon chili powder
- One teaspoon salt

Directions:

1. Wash potatoes and portion into eight slices.
2. Warm bacon fat in the microwave for 10 seconds.
3. Combine all of your dry seasonings in a bowl and toss to mix.
4. Add bacon fat to the bowl and stir.
5. Toss the wedges in the bowl and transfer to the basket.
6. Cook at the preset chicken setting, tossing halfway through.

Nutrition: Calories: 171 Sodium: 684 mg Dietary

Fiber: 5.6g Fat: 1.9g Carbs: 34.3g Protein: 5.1g

Honey Roasted Carrots

Preparation Time: 5 Minutes

Cooking Time: 10 Minutes

Servings: 4

Ingredients:

- One tablespoon olive oil
- 3 cups baby carrots
- One tablespoon honey
- salt and pepper to taste

Directions:

1. In a container, put the carrots, then using oil and honey, drizzle it.
2. Sprinkle on salt and pepper, then using a wooden spoon, blend it entirely.
3. Position the carrots in the basket, then cook at 400 degrees for 10 minutes.
4. For best results, serve immediately.

Nutrition: Calories: 83 Sodium: 74 mg Dietary Fiber: 2.5g Fat: 3.5g Carbs: 13g Protein: 1.3g

Onion Rings

Preparation Time: 7 Minutes

Cooking Time: 7 Minutes

Servings: 4

Ingredients:

- One teaspoon baking powder
- 1 cup panko breadcrumbs
- Two eggs
- One large Vidalia onion
- 1 cup all-purpose flour

Directions:

1. Peel, core, and cut the onion into rings.
2. Combine the flour, salt, and baking powder in a bag and shake well to combine.
3. Add the onions to the bag and toss to coat.
4. Beat the eggs in a shallow bowl.
5. Spread the panko crumbs over a plate.
6. Remove one ring at a Time, shake off any extra flour, dip in the egg, then dredge through the bread crumb.
7. Add 5 to 7 rings to the fryer and cook at 400 degrees for 7 minutes.

8. Flip the rings halfway through and serve hot.

Nutrition: Calories: 186 Sodium: 615 mg Dietary Fiber: 1.8g Fat: 2.6g Carbs: 33.3g Protein: 7.1g

Chicken Kebab

Preparation Time: 15 Minutes

Cooking Time: 15 Minutes

Servings: 6

Ingredients:

- Boneless Chicken Breast – 1.5 lb. cut into large, bite-sized pc
- Smoked Paprika – ½ tsp
- Turmeric – 1 tsp
- Ground Black Pepper – ½ tsp
- Plain Greek Yogurt – ¼ cup

Directions:

1. Place chicken into a large bowl.
2. Place Greek yogurt, smoked paprika, black pepper, and turmeric in a small blender container and process till you get a smooth mixture.
3. Pour the blend over the chicken and coat it evenly.
4. Allow chicken to marinate for 15 minutes.
5. Put the chicken inside the basket of the air fryer.

6. Set the air fryer to 370 degrees F and cook for 15 minutes.
7. After 8 minutes, flip the chicken over and continue cooking.
8. Once done, allow them to sit for several minutes and serve.

Nutrition: : Calories 150 Fats: 2g Protein: 20g Carbs: 0.5 g

Cinnamon Apple Chips

Preparation Time:10 minutes

Cooking Time: 8 minutes

Servings:6

Ingredients:

- 3 granny smith apples, wash, core and thinly slice
- 1tsp ground cinnamon pinch of salt

Directions:

1. Rub apple slices with cinnamon and salt and place into the air fryer basket.
2. Cook at 390 f for 8 minutes. Turn halfway through.
3. Serve and enjoy.

Nutrition: Calories: 170 Protein: 4 g. Fat: 1 g. Carbs: 6 g.

Apple Chips with Dip

Preparation Time: 10 minutes

Cooking Time: 12 minutes

Servings: 4

Ingredients:

- 1 apple, thinly slice using a mandolin slicer
- 1 tbsp almond butter
- 1/4 cup plain yogurt
- 2 tsp olive oil
- 1 tsp ground cinnamon
- Drops liquid stevia

Directions:

1. Add apple slices, oil, and cinnamon in a large bowl and toss well.
2. Spray air fryer basket with cooking spray.
3. Place apple slices in air fryer basket and cook at 375 f for 12 minutes. Turn after every 4 minutes.
4. Meanwhile, in a small bowl, mix together almond butter, yogurt, and sweetener.
5. Serve apple chips with dip and enjoy.

Nutrition: Calories 253 Total Carbs 15g Net Carbs 13g Protein 27g Fat 9g Sugar 4g Fiber 2g

Delicious Spiced Apples

Preparation Time:10 minutes

Cooking Time: 10 minutes

Servings:6

Ingredients:
- Small apples, sliced
- 1 tsp apple pie spice
- 1/2 cup erythritol
- 2 tbsp coconut oil, melted

Directions:
1. Add apple slices in a mixing bowl and sprinkle sweetener, apple pie spice, and coconut oil over apple and toss to coat.
2. Transfer apple slices in air fryer dish. Place dish in air fryer basket and cook at 350 f for 10 minutes.

Nutrition: Calories: 234 Kcal, Fat: 13.8g, Carb, 5.9g, Protein: 20g

Serve and enjoy.

Tasty Cheese Bites

Preparation Time: 10 minutes

Cooking Time: 2 minutes

Servings: 16

Ingredients:

- 8oz cream cheese, softened
- 2tbsp erythritol
- 1/2 cup almond flour
- 1/2tsp vanilla
- 4tbsp heavy cream
- 1/2cup erythritol

Directions:

1. Add cream cheese, vanilla, 1/2 cup erythritol, and 2 tbsp heavy cream in a stand mixer and mix until smooth.
2. Scoop cream cheese mixture onto the parchment lined plate and place in the refrigerator for 1 hour.
3. In a small bowl, mix together almond flour and 2 tbsp erythritol.
4. Dip cheesecake bites in remaining heavy cream and coat with almond flour mixture.

5. Place cheesecake bites in air fryer basket and air fry for 2 minutes at 350 f.
6. Make sure cheesecake bites are frozen before air fry otherwise they will melt.
7. Drizzle with chocolate syrup and serve.

Nutrition: Calories: 383 Kcal, Fat: 19.8g, Carb: 28g, Protein: 23g

Apple Chips

Preparation Time: 10 Minutes

Cooking Time: 20 Minutes

Servings: 2

Ingredients:

- 1 apple, sliced thinly
- Salt to taste
- ¼ teaspoon ground cinnamon

Directions:

1. Preheat the air fryer to 350 degrees F.
2. Toss the apple slices in salt and cinnamon.
3. Add to the air fryer.
4. Let cool before serving.

Nutrition: Calories: 59 Protein: 0.3g. Fat: 0.2g. Carbs: 15.6g.

Gooey Cinnamon Smores

Preparation Time:5 minutes | Cooking Time: 3 minutes | makes 12 s'mores

Ingredients:

- 12 whole cinnamon graham crackers, halved
- 2 (1.55-ounce) chocolate bars, cut into 12 pieces
- 12 marshmallows

Directions:

1. Arrange 12 graham cracker squares in the air fry basket in a single layer.
2. Top each square with a piece of chocolate.
3. Place the basket on the bake position.
4. Select bake, set temperature to 350ºf (180ºc), and set Time to 3 minutes.
5. After 2 minutes, remove the basket and place a marshmallow on each piece of melted chocolate. Return the basket to the air fryer grill and continue to cook for another 1 minute.
6. Remove from the air fryer grill to a serving plate.

7. Serve topped with the remaining graham cracker squares

Nutrition: Calories: 234 Kcal, Fat: 13.8g, Carb, 5.9g, Protein: 20g

Sweetened Plantains

Preparation Time: 5 Minutes

Cooking Time: 8 Minutes

Servings: 4

Ingredients:

- 2 ripe plantains, sliced
- 2 teaspoons avocado oil
- Salt to taste
- Maple syrup

Directions:

1. Toss the plantains in oil.
2. Season with salt.
3. Cook in the air fryer basket at 400 degrees F for 10 minutes, shaking after 5 minutes. Drizzle with maple syrup before serving.

Nutrition: Calories: 125 Protein: 1.2 g. Fat: 0.6 g. Carbs: 32 g.

Pear Crisp

Preparation Time: 10 Minutes

Cooking Time: 25 Minutes

Servings: 2

Ingredients:

- 1 cup flour
- 1 stick vegan butter
- 1 tablespoon cinnamon
- 1/2 cup sugar
- 2 pears, cubed

Directions:

1. Mix flour and butter to form crumbly texture.
2. Add cinnamon and sugar.
3. Put the pears in the air fryer.
4. Pour and spread the mixture on top of the pears.
5. Cook at 350 degrees F for 25 minutes.

Nutrition: Calories: 544 Protein: 7.4 g. Fat: 0.9 g. Carbs: 132.3 g.

Easy Pears Dessert

Preparation Time:10 Minutes

Cooking Time: 25 Minutes

Servings: 12

Ingredients:

- 6 big pears, cored and chopped
- 1/2 cup raisins
- 1 teaspoon ginger powder
- ¼ cup coconut sugar
- 1 teaspoon lemon zest, grated

Directions:

1. In a container that fits your air fryer, mix pears with raisins, ginger, sugar and lemon zest, stir, introduce in the fryer and cook at 350 degrees F for 25 minutes.
2. Divide into bowls and serve cold.
3. Enjoy!

Nutrition: Calories: 200 Protein: 6 g. Fat: 3 g. Carbs: 6 g.

Vanilla Strawberry Mix

Preparation Time: 10 Minutes

Cooking Time: 20 Minutes

Servings: 10

Ingredients:
- 2 tablespoons lemon juice
- 2 pounds strawberries
- 4 cups coconut sugar
- 1 teaspoon cinnamon powder
- 1 teaspoon vanilla extract

Directions:
1. In a pot that fits your air fryer, mix strawberries with coconut sugar, lemon juice, cinnamon and vanilla, stir gently, introduce in the fryer and cook at 350 degrees F for 20 minutes
2. Divide into bowls and serve cold.
3. Enjoy!

Nutrition: Calories: 140 Protein: 2 g. Fat: 0 g. Carbs: 5 g.

Sweet Bananas and Sauce

Preparation Time: 10 Minutes

Cooking Time: 20 Minutes

Servings: 4

Ingredients:

- Juice of 1/2 lemon
- 3 tablespoons agave nectar
- 1 tablespoon coconut oil
- 4 bananas, peeled and sliced diagonally
- 1/2 teaspoon cardamom seeds

Directions:

1. Arrange bananas in a pan that fits your air fryer, add agave nectar, lemon juice, oil and cardamom, introduce in the fryer and cook at 360 degrees F for 20 minutes
2. Divide bananas and sauce between plates and serve.
3. Enjoy!

Nutrition: Calories: 210 Protein: 3 g. Fat: 1 g. Carbs: 8 g.

Cinnamon Apples and Mandarin Sauce

Preparation Time: 10 Minutes

Cooking Time: 20 Minutes

Servings: 4

Ingredients:

- 4 apples, cored, peeled and cored
- 2 cups mandarin juice
- ¼ cup maple syrup
- 2 teaspoons cinnamon powder
- 1 tablespoon ginger, grated

Directions:

1. In a pot that fits your air fryer, mix apples with mandarin juice, maple syrup, cinnamon and ginger, introduce in the fryer and cook at 365 degrees F for 20 minutes
2. Divide apples mix between plates and serve warm.
3. Enjoy!

Nutrition: Calories: 170 Protein: 4 g. Fat: 1 g. Carbs: 6 g.

Cocoa Berries Cream

Preparation Time:10 Minutes

Cooking Time: 10 Minutes

Servings: 4

Ingredients:

- 3 tablespoons cocoa powder
- 14 ounces coconut cream
- 1 cup blackberries
- 1 cup raspberries
- 2 tablespoons stevia

Directions:

1. In a bowl, whisk cocoa powder with stevia and cream and stir.
2. Add raspberries and blackberries, toss gently, transfer to a pan that fits your air fryer, introduce in the fryer and cook at 350 degrees F for 10 minutes.
3. Divide into bowls and serve cold. Enjoy!

Nutrition: Calories: 205 Protein: 2 g. Fat: 34 g. Carbs: 6 g.

Sweet Vanilla Rhubarb

Preparation Time: 10 Minutes

Cooking Time: 10 Minutes

Servings: 4

Ingredients:

- 5 cups rhubarb, chopped
- 2 tablespoons coconut butter, melted
- 1/3 cup water
- 1 tablespoon stevia
- 1 teaspoon vanilla extract

Directions:

1. Put rhubarb, ghee, water, stevia and vanilla extract in a pan that fits your air fryer, introduce in the fryer and cook at 365 degrees F for 10 minutes
2. Divide into small bowls and serve cold.
3. Enjoy!

Nutrition: Calories: 103 Protein: 2 g. Fat: 2 g. Carbs: 6 g.

Cherries and Rhubarb Bowls

Preparation Time: 10 Minutes

Cooking Time: 35 Minutes

Servings: 4

Ingredients:

- 2 cups cherries, pitted and halved
- 1 cup rhubarb, sliced
- 1 cup apple juice
- 2 tablespoons sugar
- 1/2 cup raisins.

Directions:

1. In a pot that fits your air fryer, combine the cherries with the rhubarb and the other ingredients, toss, cook at 330 degrees F for 35 minutes, divide into bowls, cool down and serve.

Nutrition: Calories: 212 Protein: 7 g. Fat: 8 g. Carbs: 13 g.

Pumpkin Bowls

Preparation Time: 10 Minutes

Cooking Time: 15 Minutes

Servings: 4

Ingredients:

- 2 cups pumpkin flesh, cubed
- 1 cup heavy cream
- 1 teaspoon cinnamon powder
- 3 tablespoons sugar
- 1 teaspoon nutmeg, ground

Directions:

1. In a pot that fits your air fryer, combine the pumpkin with the cream and the other ingredients, introduce in the fryer and cook at 360 degrees F for 15 minutes.
2. Divide into bowls and serve.

Nutrition: Calories: 212 Protein: 7 g. Fat: 5 g. Carbs: 15 g.

Buttery Fennel and Garlic

Preparation Time: 10 Minutes

Cooking Time: 5 Minutes

Servings: 4

Ingredients:
- 1/2 stick butter
- 2 garlic cloves, sliced
- 1/2 teaspoon salt
- and 1/2-pounds fennel bulbs, cut into wedges
- ¼ teaspoon ground black pepper
- 1/2 teaspoon cayenne
- ¼ teaspoon dried dill weed
- 1/3 cup dry white wine
- 2/3 cup stock

Directions:
1. Set your Power XL Deluxe to Sauté mode and add butter, let it heat up
2. Add garlic and cook for 30 seconds
3. Add rest of the Ingredients:
4. Lock lid & cook on LOW pressure for 3 minutes
5. Remove lid and serve

6. Enjoy!

Nutrition: Calories: 111 Fat: 6g Saturated Fat: 2 g Carbohydrates: 2 g Fiber: 2 g Sodium: 317 mg Protein: 2 g

Lemon Mousse

Preparation Time: 10 minutes

Cooking Time: 12 minutes

Servings: 2

Ingredients:

- 4ounces cream cheese, softened
- ½ cup heavy cream
- 2tablespoons fresh lemon juice
- 2tablespoons honey
- Pinch of salt

Directions:

1. In a bowl, add all the ingredients and mix until well combined.
2. Transfer the mixture into 2 ramekins.
3. Select "Bake" of Kalorik Maxx Air Fryer Oven and then adjust the temperature to 350 degrees Fahrenheit.
4. Set the Timer for 12 minutes and press "Start/Stop" to begin cooking.
5. When the unit beeps to show that it is preheated, place the ramekins over the air rack and insert in the Kalorik Oven.

6. When cooking Time is complete, remove the ramekin from Kalorik Oven and place onto a wire rack to cool completely.
7. Refrigerate the ramekins for at least 3 hours before serving.

Nutrition: Calories 369 Total Fat 31gSaturated Fat 19.5g Cholesterol 103mg Sodium 261mg Total Carbohydrates 20g Fiber 0.1g Sugar 17.7g Protein 5.1g

Glazed Banana

Preparation Time: 10 minutes

Cooking Time: 10 minutes

Servings: 4

Ingredients:

- 2 ripe bananas, peeled and sliced lengthwise
- 1 teaspoon fresh lime juice
- 4 teaspoons maple syrup
- 1/8 teaspoon ground cinnamon

Directions:

1. Coat each banana half with lime juice.
2. Arrange the banana halves onto the greased "baking pan" cut sides up.
3. Drizzle the banana halves with maple syrup and sprinkle with cinnamon.
4. Select "Air Fry" of Kalorik Maxx Air Fryer Oven and then adjust the temperature to 350 degrees Fahrenheit.
5. Set the Timer for 10 minutes and press "Start/Stop" to begin cooking.

6. When the unit beeps to show that it is preheated, insert the baking pan in the Kalorik Oven.
7. When cooking Time is complete, remove the baking pan from Kalorik Oven and serve immediately.

Nutrition: Calories 70 Total Fat 0.2g Saturated Fat 0.1g Cholesterol 0mg Sodium 1mgTotal Carbohydrates 18g Fiber 1.6g Sugar 11.2g Protein 0.6g

Raspberry Danish

Preparation Time: 20 minutes

Cooking Time: 25 minutes

Servings: 6

Ingredients:

- 1 tube full-sheet crescent roll dough
- 4ounces cream cheese, softened
- ¼ cup raspberry jam
- ½ cup fresh raspberries, chopped
- 1 cup powdered sugar
- 2-3 tablespoons heavy whipping cream

Directions:

1. Place the sheet of crescent roll dough onto a flat surface and unroll it.
2. In a microwave-safe bowl, add the cream cheese and microwave for about 20-30 seconds.
3. Remove from microwave and stir until creamy and smooth.
4. Spread the cream cheese over the dough sheet, followed by the strawberry jam.
5. Now, place the raspberry pieces evenly across the top.

6. From the short side, roll the dough and pinch the seam to seal.
7. Arrange a greased parchment paper onto the steak tray of oven.
8. Carefully, curve the rolled pastry into a horseshoe shape and arrange onto the tray.
9. Select "Air Fry" of Kalorik Maxx Air Fryer Oven and then adjust the temperature to 350 degrees Fahrenheit.
10. Set the Timer for 25 minutes and press "Start/Stop" to begin cooking.
11. When the unit beeps to show that it is preheated, insert the tray in the Kalorik Oven.
12. When cooking Time is complete, remove the tray from Kalorik Oven and place onto a rack to cool.
13. Meanwhile, in a bowl, mix together the powdered sugar and cream.
14. Drizzle the cream mixture over cooled Danish and serve.

Nutrition: Calories 335 Total Fat 15.3g Saturated Fat 8g Cholesterol 28mg Sodium 342mg Total

Carbohydrates 45.3g Fiber 0.7g Sugar 30.1g Protein 4.4g

Blueberry Muffins

Preparation Time: 15 minutes

Cooking Time: 15 minutes

Servings: 8

Ingredients:

- ¼ cup unsweetened coconut milk
- 2 large eggs
- ½ teaspoon vanilla extract
- 1½ cups almond flour
- ¼ cup Swerve
- 1 teaspoon baking powder
- ¼ teaspoon ground cinnamon
- Pinch of ground cloves
- Pinch of ground nutmeg
- 1/8 teaspoon salt
- ½ cup fresh blueberries
- ¼ cup pecans, chopped

Directions:

1. In a blender, add the almond milk, eggs and vanilla extract and pulse for about 20-30 seconds.

2. Add the almond flour, Swerve, baking powder, spices and salt and pulse for about 30-45 seconds until well blended.
3. Transfer the mixture into a bowl
4. Gently, fold in half of the blueberries and pecans.
5. Place the mixture into 8 silicone muffin cups and top each with remaining blueberries.
6. Select "Air Fry" of Kalorik Maxx Air Fryer Oven and then adjust the temperature to 325 degrees Fahrenheit.
7. Set the Timer for 15 minutes and press "Start/Stop" to begin cooking.
8. When the unit beeps to show that it is preheated, place the cups over the air rack and insert in the Kalorik Oven.
9. When cooking Time is complete, remove the cups from Kalorik Oven and place onto a wire rack to cool for about 10 minutes.
10. Carefully, invert the muffins onto the wire rack to completely cool before serving.

Nutrition: Calories 191 Total Fat 16.5g Saturated Fat 3g Cholesterol 47mg Sodium 54mg Total

Carbohydrates 14.8g Fiber 3.2g Sugar 9.7g Protein 6.8g

Cranberry Cupcakes

Preparation Time: 15 minutes

Cooking Time: 15 minutes

Servings: 10

Ingredients:

- 4½ ounces self-rising flour
- ½ teaspoon baking powder
- Pinch of salt
- ½ ounce cream cheese, softened
- 4¾ ounces butter, softened
- 4¼ ounces caster sugar
- 2 eggs
- 2 teaspoons fresh lemon juice
- ½ cup fresh cranberries

Directions:

1. In a bowl, mix together the flour, baking powder, and salt.
2. In another bowl, mix together the cream cheese, and butter.
3. Add the sugar and beat until fluffy and light.
4. Add the eggs, one at a Time and whisk until just combined.

5. Add the flour mixture and stir until well combined.
6. Stir in the lemon juice.
7. Place the mixture into silicone cups and top each with cranberries evenly, pressing slightly.
8. Select "Air Fry" of Kalorik Maxx Air Fryer Oven and then adjust the temperature to 365 degrees Fahrenheit.
9. Set the Timer for 15 minutes and press "Start/Stop" to begin cooking.
10. When the unit beeps to show that it is preheated, place the cups over the air rack and insert in the Kalorik Oven.
11. When cooking Time is complete, remove the cups from Kalorik Oven and place onto a wire rack to cool for about 10 minutes.
12. Carefully, invert the cupcakes onto the wire rack to completely cool before serving.

Nutrition: Calories 209 Total Fat 12.4g Saturated Fat 7.5g Cholesterol 63mg Sodium 110mg Total Carbohydrates 22.6g Fiber 0.6g Sugar 12.4g Protein 2.7g

Zucchini Mug Cake

Preparation Time: 10 minutes

Cooking Time: 20 minutes

Servings: 1

Ingredients:

- ¼ cup whole-wheat pastry flour
- 1 tablespoon sugar
- ¼ teaspoon baking powder
- ¼ teaspoon ground cinnamon
- Pinch of salt
- 2 tablespoons plus 2 teaspoons milk
- 2 tablespoons zucchini, grated and squeezed
- 2 tablespoons almonds, chopped
- 1 tablespoon raisins
- 2 teaspoons maple syrup

Directions:

1. In a bowl, mix together the flour, sugar, baking powder, cinnamon and salt.
2. Add the remaining ingredients and mix until well combined.

3. Place the mixture into a lightly greased ramekin.
4. Select "Bake" of Kalorik Maxx Air Fryer Oven and then adjust the temperature to 350 degrees Fahrenheit.
5. Set the Timer for 20 minutes and press "Start/Stop" to begin cooking.
6. When the unit beeps to show that it is preheated, place the ramekin over the air rack and insert in the Kalorik Oven.
7. When cooking Time is complete, remove the ramekin from Kalorik Oven and place onto a wire rack to cool slightly before serving.

Nutrition: Calories 310 Total Fat 7g Saturated Fat 0.9g Cholesterol 3mg Sodium 175mg Total Carbohydrates 57.5g Fiber 3.2g Sugar 27.5g Protein 7.2g

Chocolate Brownies

Preparation Time:15 minutes

Cooking Time: 15 minutes

Servings: 4

Ingredients:

- ½ cup all-purpose flour
- ¾ cup sugar
- 6tablespoons cacao powder
- ¼ teaspoon baking powder
- ¼ teaspoon salt
- ¼ cup butter, melted
- 2large eggs
- 1 tablespoon olive oil
- ½ teaspoon pure vanilla extract

Directions:

1. Grease a 7-inch baking dish generously. Set aside.
2. In a bowl, add all the ingredients and mix until well combined.
3. Place the mixture into the baking dish and with the back of a spoon, smooth the top surface.

4. Arrange the baking pan of oven in the bottom of Kalorik Digital Air Fryer Oven.
5. Select "Air Fry" of Kalorik Maxx Air Fryer Oven and then adjust the temperature to 320 degrees Fahrenheit.
6. Set the Timer for 30 minutes and press "Start/Stop" to begin cooking.
7. When the unit beeps to show that it is preheated, place the baking dish over the baking pan and insert in the Kalorik Oven.
8. When cooking Time is complete, remove the pan from Kalorik Oven and place onto a wire rack to cool completely before cutting.
9. Cut the brownie into desired-sized squares and serve.

Nutrition: Calories 367 Total Fat 19.2g Saturated Fat 9.5g Cholesterol 124mg Sodium 265mg Total Carbohydrates 53.6g Fiber 2.7g Sugar 37.8g Protein 6.4g

Apple Crisp

Preparation Time: 15 minutes

Cooking Time: 40 minutes

Servings: 2

Ingredients:

- 1½ cups apple, peeled, cored and sliced
- ¼ cup sugar, divided
- 1½ teaspoons cornstarch
- 3 tablespoons all-purpose flour
- ¼ teaspoon ground cinnamon
- Pinch of salt
- 1½ tablespoons cold butter, chopped
- 3 tablespoons rolled oats

Directions:

1. In a bowl, place apple slices, 1 teaspoon of sugar and cornstarch and toss to coat well.
2. Divide the plum mixture into lightly greased 2 (8-ounce) ramekins.
3. In a bowl, mix together the flour, remaining sugar, cinnamon and salt.
4. With 2 forks, blend in the butter until a crumbly mixture form.
5. Add the oats and gently, stir to combine.

6. Place the oat mixture over apple slices into each ramekin.
7. Select "Bake" of Kalorik Maxx Air Fryer Oven and then adjust the temperature to 350 degrees Fahrenheit.
8. Set the Timer for 40 minutes and press "Start/Stop" to begin cooking.
9. When the unit beeps to show that it is preheated, place the ramekins over the air rack and insert in the Kalorik Oven.
10. When cooking Time is complete, remove the ramekins from Kalorik Oven and place onto a wire rack to cool for about 10 minutes before serving.

Nutrition: Calories 337 Total Fat 9.6g Saturated Fat 5.6g Cholesterol 23mg Sodium 141mg Total Carbohydrates 64.3g Fiber 5.3g Sugar 42.5gProtein 2.8g

Lightning Source UK Ltd.
Milton Keynes UK
UKHW022023240621
386092UK00002BA/308